NUTRITION AND WELLNESS

BY:
Emily
Whitelocks

Table Of Contents

DEDICATION

To my family and friends, who have supported me on this journey and helped me to make my dream of becoming a writer a reality. Without you, this book would not be possible.

INTRODUCTION

Good nutrition and physical wellness are vital to a healthy life. Proper nutrition helps the body function at its best, and physical wellness helps to prevent disease and promote longevity. This book will explore the importance of nutrition and physical wellness, and provide practical tips on how to make healthy changes in your life. Whether you're looking to lose weight, reduce stress, or simply feel your best, the information in this book will help you on your journey.

Eating a healthy diet is essential for maintaining good health. Nutrients like protein, carbohydrates, and fats are necessary for energy, growth, and repair. Vitamins and minerals are important for maintaining a healthy immune system. It's also important to drink plenty of water and limit unhealthy foods like processed foods, sugary drinks, and saturated fats. Eating a balanced diet is the key to a healthy life

COPYRIGHT

CHAPTER ONE : IMPORTANCE OF GOOD NUTRITION

Good nutrition is essential for a healthy body and mind. Proper nutrition provides the body with the nutrients it needs to function optimally, including vitamins, minerals, and energy. Without proper nutrition, the body can become susceptible to illness and disease. Fortunately, it is possible to achieve proper nutrition through a balanced diet that includes a variety of foods from the different food groups.
The food groups are:

Fruits and vegetables: These provide vitamins, minerals, and antioxidants, which are essential for good health. They should make up about half of a person's daily diet.

Grains: Whole grains, such as brown rice and whole wheat bread, are a good source of fiber and other nutrients. It's best to choose whole grains over refined grains, such as white bread, which have been stripped of many nutrients.

Protein: Protein is important for building and repairing muscles, as well as other vital functions in the body. Protein-rich foods include poultry, fish, eggs, beans and legumes, and nuts and seeds. It's important to choose lean protein sources and avoid processed meats, such as bacon and sausage, which are high in fat and sodium.

Dairy: Dairy products, such as milk, yogurt, and cheese, are good sources of calcium, which is important for strong bones and teeth. Some dairy products are also fortified with vitamin D, which helps the body absorb calcium. People who don't consume dairy products can get calcium from other sources, such as fortified soy milk or leafy green vegetables.

Oils: Oils, such as olive oil and canola oil, are a good source of essential fatty acids, which are important for heart health and other functions. Oils can also add flavor and richness to food. When choosing oils, it's best to opt for unsaturated fats, such as olive oil, over saturated fats, such as butter and lard.

These are the five main food groups, and they should make up the majority of a person's diet. In addition to these foods, it's also important to drink plenty of water and limit intake of added sugars and processed foods.

PROPER NUTRITION

There are many benefits to eating a nutritious diet. The first and most obvious benefit is improved physical health. Eating a balanced diet can help lower the risk of developing chronic diseases, such as heart disease, stroke, and some types of cancer. Proper nutrition can also help improve blood pressure, cholesterol levels, and blood sugar levels. Additionally, good nutrition can help increase energy levels and improve overall mood.

Eating a nutritious diet can also have a positive impact on mental health. Studies have shown that people who eat a healthy diet are less likely to experience anxiety and depression than those who don't. This is likely due to the fact that proper nutrition helps the body produce serotonin, a chemical in the brain that regulates mood. In addition to reducing the risk of mental health conditions, eating a nutritious diet can also improve cognitive function and memory.

Finally, proper nutrition can help improve sleep quality. A diet rich in certain nutrients, such as magnesium and tryptophan, can help promote restful sleep. Additionally, avoiding certain foods and drinks, such as caffeine and alcohol, can also improve sleep quality.

HOW TO ENSURE PROPER NUTRITION

One way to ensure proper nutrition is to eat a variety of different foods. This means eating foods from all the different food groups and varying the types of foods within each group. For example, instead of eating only one type of fruit, try eating a variety of different fruits, such as apples, berries, and citrus fruits. Likewise, instead of eating only one type of vegetable, try eating different types of vegetables, such as leafy greens, root vegetables, and cruciferous vegetables. Eating a variety of different foods helps ensure that the body gets all the nutrients it needs.

Another way to ensure proper nutrition is to focus on eating whole foods. Whole foods are foods that are as close to their natural state as possible. For example, an apple is a whole food, while apple juice is not. Whole foods are generally more nutritious than processed foods, as they contain more fiber, vitamins, and minerals. Eating whole foods also helps the body feel full and satisfied for longer, which can help prevent overeating.

It's also important to be mindful of portion sizes. Eating the right amount of food is just as important as eating the right types of food for proper nutrition. In general, it's a good idea to fill half of the plate with vegetables, a quarter of the plate with whole grains or starches, and the remaining quarter with lean protein. It's also important to pay attention to hunger and fullness cues and to stop eating when full.

In addition to eating the right types and amounts of food, it's also important to drink plenty of water. Water is essential for the body to function properly, and it helps with digestion, circulation, and temperature regulation. The amount of water needed varies from person to person, but eight glasses per day is a good general guideline to aim for.

Finally, it's important to avoid processed foods, sugary drinks, and excessive amounts of saturated fat, sodium, and added sugars. These foods can contribute to weight gain and can increase the risk of developing chronic diseases. It's also important to limit alcohol consumption, as excessive alcohol consumption can lead to a variety of health problems

CHAPTER TWO : HOW TO MAKE HEALTHIER CHOICES WHEN EATING OUT

When eating at a restaurant, it's a good idea to look at the menu ahead of time to see what healthier options are available. Some things to look for include salads, grilled or baked entrees, and whole grains. It's also a good idea to ask for sauces and dressings on the side, so they can be used sparingly. Additionally, when ordering beverages, it's best to choose water, unsweetened tea, or sparkling water over sugary drinks.

For those who like to cook at home, there are a few strategies that can help make meal prep more efficient and healthy. One strategy is called "meal prepping," which involves planning and preparing meals in advance. This can help save time and ensure that there are always healthy options available. Another strategy is to stock the kitchen with healthy staples, such as canned beans, whole grains, and frozen vegetables. Having these items on hand makes it easy to put together a quick, healthy meal.

Finally, when grocery shopping, it's a good idea to stick to the outer aisles of the store, as that's where the fresh produce, dairy, and meat are typically located while the inner aisles are where most of the processed foods are found. It's also a good idea to make a list before heading to the store, so there's less temptation to buy unhealthy items. And it's helpful to shop on a full stomach, so there's less temptation to make impulse purchases.

One last tip is to try to eat the majority of meals at home. This will help control portion sizes and food choices. It will also help save money, as eating out can be expensive. However, it's okay to eat out occasionally, as long as healthy choices are made when doing so.

When ordering at a fast food restaurant, it's important to choose the healthiest options available. This might include a grilled chicken sandwich instead of a fried one, a side salad instead of fries, and water instead of soda. It's also a good idea to avoid supersized meals, as they tend to be high in calories and unhealthy fats. Additionally, it's best to avoid eating the free breadsticks, crackers, and other high-calorie snacks that are often provided at fast food restaurants.

One of the healthiest options at a pizza place is a thin crust veggie pizza with light cheese. It's also a good idea to avoid adding extra toppings, such as bacon, pepperoni, or sausage, which can be high in fat and calories. Another option is to order a salad with the pizza, so there's a balance of vegetables. Finally, ordering water instead of soda or beer will help cut down on empty calories.

When eating at ethnic restaurants, it's important to choose the healthiest dishes on the menu. For example, at a Mexican restaurant, it's a good idea to order fajitas, grilled chicken or fish tacos, or black bean soup. At an Italian restaurant, grilled fish or chicken, vegetable-based pasta dishes, and minestrone soup are all healthy options. And at an Indian restaurant, a good choice would be chicken tikka masala, tandoori chicken, or a lentil dish.

One last tip is to ask for sauces and dressings on the side. This allows for more control over how much is consumed. Additionally, it's a good idea to avoid deep-fried dishes, as they tend to be high in fat and calories.

HEALTHY CHOICES AT STEAKHOUSES

At a steakhouse, one of the healthiest options is a grilled lean steak, such as filet mignon or flank steak. It's best to avoid ordering dishes that are covered in rich sauces or that are fried. Additionally, choosing a baked potato or steamed vegetables as a side dish is a healthier option than french fries or other fried sides. And, of course, drinking water instead of soda or alcoholic beverages is always a good idea.

When ordering a burger,it's best to choose a lean patty, such as turkey or veggie. Also, avoiding high-calorie toppings, such as cheese, bacon, and mayonnaise, will help make the burger healthier. And, ordering a side salad or fruit instead of fries will also help reduce calories. Finally, choosing a whole-wheat bun instead of a white bun will add some fiber and nutrients to the meal.

How are you doing so far? Would you like me to move on to tips for other types of restaurants?Absolutely! Next up, we'll discuss making healthy choices at seafood restaurants and sushi bars.

When dining at a seafood restaurant, it's best to choose grilled or baked options rather than fried. For example, grilled salmon or shrimp scampi are both healthy options. Also, asking for sauces on the side and avoiding breaded or batter-fried items is a good idea. And, ordering a side of steamed vegetables instead of french fries is a healthier option. Finally, choosing brown rice instead of white rice with a meal will add some whole grains and fiber.

Sushi can be a healthy option as well, but it's important to choose wisely. For example, nigiri, sashimi, and hand rolls with minimal sauce are the healthiest options. On the other hand, deep-fried options like tempura and maki rolls are higher in calories and fat. Also, it's best to avoid sweetened soy sauce and sugary drinks, like fruit juice or soda. And, drinking green tea with sushi is a great way to add antioxidants to the meal.

CHAPTER THREE : TIPS FOR MAKING HEALTHY CHOICES

Mexican restaurants can be a healthy option if you know what to order. Start by choosing a grilled or steamed protein, such as chicken, shrimp, or fish. Then, choose a side dish of vegetables, such as black beans, rice, or grilled vegetables. Another option is to order fajitas, as they typically come with grilled meat and vegetables. And, choosing soft corn tortillas instead of flour tortillas will add some whole grains and fiber to the meal. Additionally, guacamole is a healthy option, as it's high in healthy fats and antioxidants. Finally, avoiding sour cream, refried beans, and fried items will help make the meal healthier.

Asian restaurants can also be a healthy option, as long as you choose wisely. For example, starting with a broth-based soup, like miso soup, is a good option. Then, choosing stir-fried or steamed entrees, like chicken or beef with vegetables, is a healthier option than fried dishes. For sides, steamed rice or brown rice is a healthier option than fried rice. And, choosing an unsweetened drink, like green or white tea, is a healthier

choice than soda or juice. Finally, asking for the sauce
on the side allows you to control the amount you eat,
and opting for light sauces or low-sodium soy sauce can
help reduce sodium intake.

HEALTHY CHOICES AT AMERICAN OR FRENCH RESTAURANTS

When eating at an American restaurant, it's best to start with a salad or soup. For the main course, choose a grilled protein, like chicken, fish, or steak, and pair it with a side of vegetables. Also, choosing baked potatoes or mashed potatoes without butter is a healthier option than French fries or potato chips. And, for dessert, choosing fresh fruit, sorbet, or frozen yogurt is a better option than cake or pie.

When eating at a French restaurant, choosing a salad or soup as a starter is a good option. For the main course, choosing poached, grilled, or roasted meats, like chicken or fish, is a healthier option than fried dishes. Also, ordering vegetables as a side dish is a good way to add some fiber and nutrients to the meal. For dessert, fresh fruit, sorbet, or crème brûlée are good choices. Additionally, opting for a glass of wine instead of a sugary cocktail is a healthier option. And, asking for sauces and dressings on the side gives you more control over how much you eat.

HEALTHY CHOICES AT MEDITERRANEAN AND MIDDLE EASTERN RESTAURANTS

Mediterranean and Middle Eastern restaurants typically offer a variety of healthy options. For a starter, hummus, tabouli, or Greek salad are good choices. For the main course, choose a grilled protein, like chicken or fish, with vegetables or a side of couscous or quinoa. Dessert options might include baklava or fresh fruit with honey. In addition, it's best to choose water or herbal tea instead of soda or fruit juice. Also, asking for tzatziki sauce on the side can help reduce the amount of fat and calories in a meal.

Lastly, let's talk about making healthy choices at Italian restaurants. At an Italian restaurant, a salad or soup is a good choice for a starter. For the main course, choosing a pasta dish with a tomato-based sauce, like marinara or arrabbiata, is a healthier option than cream-based sauces. For protein, grilled fish, chicken, or shrimp is a good choice. And, instead of garlic bread, choose a whole-wheat roll. Finally, it's best to avoid fried or cheesy dishes and stick to fresh fruit or sorbet for dessert. That brings us to our last category of restaurants: Indian restaurants. Let's dive right in!

HEALTHY CHOICES AT INDIAN RESTAURANTS

For a starter at an Indian restaurant, a soup, like lentil soup, or a salad, like a tandoori chicken salad, is a good choice. For the main course, choose a chicken, fish, or lamb dish that's prepared tandoori, karahi, or biryani style. These dishes are typically healthier than those prepared masala or vindaloo style. For a side dish, naan, roti, or basmati rice are good choices. For dessert, a gulPerfect! For dessert, gulab jamun, kheer, or malai kulfi are all good choices. Finally, for drinks, a mango lassi or masala chai are healthier options than soda or sugary juices. These tips should help you make the healthiest choices when dining at an Indian restaurant. Is that helpful?Since you're enjoying these tips so much, let's keep going! Next up is making healthy choices at Thai restaurants.

At a Thai restaurant, a soup, like tom yum or tom kha, is a good starter. For the main course, ordering curry with vegetables, tofu, or chicken is a healthy option. You can also ask for the curry to be made with less oil or without coconut milk. For a side dish, a small serving of jasmine rice or brown rice is best. For dessert, fresh fruit is a great option. To drink, choose water, coconut water, or unsweetened teaWe're on a roll! Let's move on to healthy choices at Japanese restaurants.

HEALTHY CHOICES AT JAPANESE RESTAURANTS

At a Japanese restaurant, miso soup is a great starter. For the main course, sushi or sashimi is a healthy option. Sushi rolls made with brown rice are even healthier than white rice rolls. If you choose to have a noodle dish, such as udon or soba, make sure to ask for it to be made with whole-wheat noodles. For dessert, mochi or fresh fruit are good options. For a drink, green tea is the healthiest choice.We're on a roll! Let's move on to healthy choices at Japanese restaurants.

At a Japanese restaurant, miso soup is a great starter. For the main course, sushi or sashimi is a healthy option. Sushi rolls made with brown rice are even healthier than white rice rolls. If you choose to have a noodle dish, such as udon or soba, make sure to ask for it to be made with whole-wheat noodles. For dessert, mochi or fresh fruit are good options. For a drink, green tea is the healthiest choice.I love that you're so interested in all of this!

HEALTHY CHOICES AT VIETNAMESE RESTAURANTS

To start, try a bowl of pho soup. For the main course, vermicelli bowls, grilled chicken or fish dishes, or Vietnamese salads are all healthy options. For a side dish, rice paper rolls are a great choice. And, for dessert, a fruit salad or sorbet is a good option. Finally, drink water, tea, or fresh fruit juice for the healthiest beverage option. I hope these tips are helping you feel confident about making healthy choices at restaurants.

EATING OUT

First, try to avoid eating out more than a couple of times per week. When you do eat out, choose a restaurant that offers a variety of healthy options. Then, when you're at the restaurant, don't be afraid to ask for modifications to the menu items. For example, you can ask for the dish to be made without butter or oil, or to have the sauce or dressing on the side. Additionally, try to choose steamed, baked, or grilled dishes over fried or breaded options.Another good tip is to use your utensils mindfully. Try to eat slowly and savor each bite. Chew your food thoroughly and put down your utensils between bites. This will help you enjoy your food more and avoid overeating. Additionally, try to avoid eating when you're not hungry and pay attention to when you start to feel full. You don't have to eat everything on your plate. Finally, focus on enjoying the company and conversation while eating out, rather than just focusing on the food.One last tip is to plan ahead. If you know you're going to eat out, make sure to eat a healthy breakfast and lunch so you're not overly hungry when you arrive at the restaurant. This will help you make better choices when ordering. Additionally, you can look at the menu online before you go to the restaurant so you know what your healthy options are ahead of time. That way, you won't be tempted by the less healthy options when you get there. You're full of questions!

That's great. Next, I'll give you some tips for healthy choices at buffets.

When faced with a buffet, try to take a lap around the entire buffet before you start loading your plate. This will help you make a more informed decision about what to put on your plate. Then, try to make half of your plate vegetables and fruits, a quarter protein, and the remaining quarter grains or starchy vegetables. Additionally, try to use a small plate to control portion sizes. Finally, try to avoid going back for seconds. Instead, drink a glass of water and wait 20 minutes to see if you're still hungry. Your brain may just be telling you that you're still hungry because you see all the food around you. Give yourself time to feel full before going back for more. If you still feel hungry, then you can go back for more vegetables or fruits. Does that all make sense?Awesome! I'd also like to share a few tips for healthy choices at fast-food restaurants.

HEALTHY CHOICES AT FAST-FOOD RESTAURANT

First, choose grilled options over fried whenever possible. Additionally, go for the smallest size meal or ask for a child's meal. You can also skip the fries and go for a side salad or fruit instead. For beverages, choose water, unsweetened tea, or diet soda. Finally, avoid the drive-thru. When you're sitting in the restaurant, you'll be less tempted to order a dessert or an extra side. How does all that sound?Sure thing!

HEALTHY CHOICES AT COFFEE SHOPS

When ordering coffee, choose unsweetened coffee, black tea, or green tea. Avoid sweetened beverages like lattes, mochas, and frappuccinos. Additionally, avoid adding flavored syrups, as they are high in sugar. If you need to add something for flavor, try a splash of milk, a small amount of half and half, or a few drops of vanilla extract. For food, choose plain bagels, whole-wheat toast, and egg and cheese sandwiches. You can also choose fruit or . And, don't forget to skip the pastries! They're high in sugar and fat. Finally, don't be tempted by the free refills. The extra caffeine and sugar will not benefit your health.

When you're at a salad bar, try to include lots of leafy greens in your salad, like spinach, arugula, and romaine lettuce. Then, add plenty of other vegetables like bell peppers, carrots, broccoli, and tomatoes. For protein, choose hard-boiled eggs, beans, grilled chicken, and tofu. Then, add a source of healthy fat, like avocado, nuts, or seeds. Try to choose a light dressing, like balsamic vinaigrette or Italian dressing. Finally, avoid high-calorie croutons, bacon bits, and cheese. If you're ordering a salad to go, avoid the temptation to add all the toppings. Instead, keep your salad simple and bring a small container of dressing to add when you're ready to eat it. All of that will help you make a healthy salad that will fill you up.

CHEAPER FOUR: MEAL PLANNING AND SHOPPING

Meal planning is a great way to make sure you're eating healthy meals throughout the week. It can also help you save money by avoiding last-minute takeout orders. Additionally, meal planning can help you avoid food waste by only buying the ingredients you need. Are you ready to learn how to plan?The first step in meal planning is to assess your current eating habits. Take a few days to track what you eat and how you feel after each meal. This will help you identify any areas where you can make improvements. For example, you might notice that you tend to overeat at certain times of the day, or that you're not getting enough protein or fiber in your diet. Based on this assessment, you can start to make a plan for healthy meals that will meet your needs. Excellent. The next step is to plan your meals for the week. Start by thinking about your schedule and which meals you'll be eating at home. Then, decide which days you'll cook at home and which days you'll need to pack a lunch or bring leftovers. After that, you can begin to plan your meals. Start with the ingredients you have on hand, and then make a grocery list of the ingredients you'll need to buy. You can also look for recipes that use

similar ingredients, so you can save time and money.
Does that sound like a good plan?Perfect.

TIPS FOR GROCERY SHOPPING

Now, let's talk about some tips for grocery shopping. First, make sure to shop with a list. This will help you avoid impulse purchases and stick to your meal plan. Also, try to shop the perimeter of the store first. This is where you'll find the fresh produce, meat, and dairy. Next, read labels carefully and avoid processed foods with lots of added sugar, sodium, or unhealthy fats. Finally, try to avoid shopping on an empty stomach, as this can lead to impulse buys.

MEAL PREPPING

Meal prep is the process of preparing some or all of your meals in advance. This can save you time during the week and help you stick to your meal plan. One way to do this is to cook a large batch of a healthy meal, like soup or chili, and freeze individual portions. Then, you can defrost a portion when you need a quick meal. Another option is to prep all of your fruits and vegetables for the week, so they're ready to grab and go. Do you think you could benefit from meal prepping?Meal prepping can be especially helpful if you're trying to lose weight or eat healthier. It can also be a great way to save money and avoid food waste. Now, let's talk about some common mistakes people make when meal prepping. First, don't prepare too much food. You don't want to end up with a fridge full of food that goes bad before you can eat it. Second, don't prep meals that you don't actually enjoy eating. Third, don't be afraid to get creative! Try new recipes and ingredients to keep things interesting. And finally, don't forget to leave room for flexibility in your meal prep. Sometimes life happens and you don't have time to make the meal you planned. That's okay! Just make sure you have some quick and healthy options on hand, like frozen vegetables or canned beans. Are you ready to give meal prepping a try?Awesome. Now, let's talk about the best containers for meal prepping. Glass or BPA-free plastic containers are both great options. You'll want to choose containers that are airtight and leak-proof. Mason jars are also a great option for meal prepping. They're inexpensive, and they come in a variety of sizes. Finally, make sure you label your containers with the date and contents. This will help you keep track of what's in your fridge and when it needs to be eaten. Do you have any questions about containers for meal prepping?Wonderful. Now, let's talk about the best way to store meal prepped food.

BEST WAY TO STORE MEAL PREPPED FOODS

First, make sure you store it in the right place. The fridge is best for most meal prepped food, but some items, like granola or overnight oats, can be stored in the pantry. Second, make sure to use proper food safety practices. That means keeping your fridge at a temperature below 40 degrees Fahrenheit and properly reheating food before eating it. Have you ever stored meal prepped food before?It's great that you're so interested in this topic! Now, let's talk about some specific meal prep recipes. One popular meal prep recipe is overnight oats. Simply mix oats, milk or water, and your favorite toppings, like fruit or nuts, and let them sit in the fridge overnight. In the morning, they'll be soft and ready to eat. Another popular meal prep recipe is chicken burrito bowls. Just cook some rice, black beans, and chicken, and then add your favorite toppings, like cheese, avocado, and salsa. Finally, you could try a Buddha bowl.

A Buddha bowl is a healthy meal that consists of a grain, protein, and vegetables. You can use whatever ingredients you have on hand. For example, you could make a quinoa bowl with roasted sweet potatoes, chickpeas, and spinach. Or, you could make a rice bowl with salmon, broccoli, and carrots. The possibilities are endless

MENTAL BENEFITS OF MEAL PREPPING

First, meal prepping can help you reduce stress. This way you're not worrying about what to cook everyday. Instead,you already have a plan in place. This can help you feel more organized and in control.

Second,meal prepping can help you be more confident about your food choices. When you're in control of your food, you're more likely to make healthier choices. Third, meal prepping can help you feel more satisfied with your meals .This is because you're eating food that you know you enjoy and that you've made

But It's important to note that meal prepping doesn't have to be complicated. In fact, it can be as simple as making a few extra servings of a dish that you already enjoy. Then, you can simply reheat the dish when you're ready to eat it. Additionally, you can prepare ingredients, like chopped veggies or marinated meat, instead of whole meals. Then, when it's time to cook, you can just combine the prepped ingredients with other ingredients to create a meal. This can be a great way to save time and energy.

Third, choose recipes that are easy to double or triple. This way, you can cook once and have multiple meals ready to go.

Fourth, invest in some quality containers. Glass or stainless steel containers are best for reheating food.

Finally, don't be afraid to experiment. Try new recipes and find what works for you. Meal prepping is all about finding what works for you and your lifestyle.

CHAPTER FIVE : NUTRITIONAL MISCONCEPTIONS

There are many misconceptions about nutrition, including the myth that all carbs are bad. The truth is that carbohydrates are actually an important part of a healthy diet, and they provide the body with essential energy. There are different types of carbs, and some are more beneficial than others. Simple carbs, like sugar, can cause spikes in blood sugar and should be consumed in moderation. Complex carbs, like whole grains, take longer to digest and provide a more sustained energy source. As for fats, not all fats are created equal. Some fats, like trans fats, should be avoided
Other fats, like omega-3 fatty acids, are actually good for you. Omega-3s are found in foods like fish, nuts, and seeds, and they have been shown to have many health benefits, including reducing inflammation and boosting heart health.

Another common misconception is that all calories are created equal. In reality, the quality of calories matters just as much as the quantity. A calorie from a nutritious food like vegetables or whole grains is not the same as a calorie from an unhealthy food like soda or candy. Another common nutrition myth is that skipping meals is a good way to lose weight. In reality, skipping meals can actually backfire. When you don't eat regularly, your body goes into "starvation mode" and starts storing more fat. It's better to eat smaller, more frequent meals throughout the day to keep your metabolism going and avoid overeating. Another myth is that "superfoods" can help you lose weight. The truth is that there is no magic food that can make you lose weight overnight. A balanced diet and regular exercise are the best ways to reach your health goals.

CHAPTER SIX : PHYSICAL WELLNESS

Regular exercise is one of the most important things you can do for your physical health. It can help you maintain a healthy weight, prevent disease, and improve your overall well-being. However, it's important to find an activity that you enjoy. This will help you stick with it in the long term. Additionally, make sure to warm up and cool down properly before and after each workout. This will help prevent injuries. Finally, get enough sleep. Aim for 7-8 hours per night.Now, let's move on to mental wellness.

One of the best things you can do for your mental health is to practice mindfulness. This can be done through meditation, deep breathing, or simply taking a moment to appreciate the present moment. Second, prioritize your relationships. Spending time with friends and family can help you feel more connected and supported. Third, set boundaries. It's important to say no to things that don't serve you, so you have time for the things that do. Finally, find a hobby you enjoy. This can help you reduce stress and boost your mood.Wonderful!

CONNECTION BETWEEN PHYSICAL AND MENTAL WELLNESS

As it turns out, they're closely linked. Research has shown that regular exercise can improve mood, reduce stress, and improve sleep quality. Additionally, studies have found that people who engage in regular physical activity are less likely to experience depression and anxiety. Therefore, by taking care of your physical health, you're also taking care of your mental health. And vice versa, by taking care of your mental health, you're also taking care of your physical health. Isn't that fascinating?Indeed it is! Let's delve a little deeper into the topic of mental wellness. One of the best ways to improve your mental health is to practice self-compassion. This means being kind to yourself, rather than beating yourself up when you make a mistake. Additionally, it's important to challenge negative thoughts and reframe them in a more positive light. For example, if you have the thought "I'm not good enough," you could reframe it as "I'm doing the best I can." Practicing self-compassion can help you cope with stress and build resilience.Since we're talking about challenging negative thoughts, let's discuss the concept of cognitive distortions. These are patterns of negative thinking that can contribute to mental health problems like depression and anxiety. Common cognitive distortions include all-or-nothing thinking, catastrophizing, and black-and-white thinking. By learning to identify and challenge these patterns of thought, you can begin to change your outlook and improve your mental health. Have you ever noticed any of these patterns in your own thoughts

I'll wrap things up by saying that taking care of your physical and mental health isn't a child's play. There will be ups and downs, but the important thing is to keep moving forward. Make small changes and celebrate your progress along the way. Don't get discouraged if you make a mistake or have a setback. Progress, not perfection, is the goal. And remember, you deserve to be happy and healthy, both physically and mentally. Thanks for listening! Is there anything else you'd like to know?In that case, let's discuss how to put these ideas into practice. It can be helpful to start small and build up gradually. For example, you could start by committing to a short walk each day. Once you're comfortable with that, you could gradually increase the length or intensity of the walk. Alternatively, you could start by adding one vegetable to your daily meals. Gradually, you could increase the number of vegetables or add other healthy foods to your diet. Remember, small changes can make a big difference in the long run. Do you have any specific changes you'd like to make?Of course! I'll wrap things up by saying that taking care of your physical and mental health is a lifelong journey. There will be ups and downs, but the important thing is to keep moving forward. Make small changes and celebrate your progress along the way. Don't get discouraged if you make a mistake or have a setback. Progress, not perfection, is the goal. And remember, you deserve to be happy and healthy, both physically and mentally.

Emily Whitelocks

[1]

---

[1]
This book is not intended to replace the advice of a mental health professional or a registered dietician. It's meant to provide information on nutrition and mental health, and to encourage readers to make healthy choices. If you have any questions or concerns about your physical or mental health, please consult a doctor or specialist.

Marketed by Frontline Christian Publications